Miscarriage after Infertility

Miscarriage
after
Infertility

A Woman's Guide to Coping

Margaret Comerford Freda, RN
and Carrie F. Semelsberger, RN

Fairview Press
Minneapolis

MISCARRIAGE AFTER INFERTILITY

Published by Fairview Press, 2450 Riverside Avenue, Minneapolis, Minnesota 55454. Fairview Press is a division of Fairview Health Services, a community-focused health system affiliated with the University of Minnesota and providing a complete range of services, from the prevention of illness and injury to care for the most complex medical conditions. For a free current catalog of Fairview Press titles, please call toll-free 1-800-544-8207. Or visit our Web site at www.fairviewpress.org.

Library of Congress Cataloging-in-Publication Data
Freda, Margaret Comerford.
Miscarriage after infertility : a woman's guide to coping / Margaret Comerford Freda, Carrie F. Semelsberger.
    p. cm.
    ISBN 1-57749-132-7
      1. Miscarriage—Popular works. 2. Fertility, Human—Popular works.
    I. Semelsberger, Carrie F., 1973- II. Title.
    RG648.F725 2003
    618.3'92--dc21

First Printing: September 2003

Printed in the United States of America
08 07 06 05 04 03   7 6 5 4 3 2 1

Cover by Laurie Ingram Design (www.laurieingramdesign.com)
Interior by Corey Sevett, Artisan Creative Computer Services

Acknowledgments

MCF: For Kit, a great nurse who found the women we interviewed and was of such incredible assistance. For the women who shared their stories and helped us to understand. For Nanette, who never gave up hope and was always encouraging. For Cheryl, who so generously shared her expertise. For my youngest daughter, who wondered why she was given the cross to bear, and then found out. For John, the best of all men. For Alyse, who couldn't put it down and encouraged us to continue. For AGS, the pot of gold at the end of the rainbow.

CFS: To Dave—thank you for being the amazing man you are . . . your unending support means everything to me. You are my true love and my forever partner. To my parents and my sister—I'll never be able to thank you enough for your unconditional support, which has seen me through good times and bad. And to Abby, for your outstanding disposition and your infectious smile—you bring such joy to my each and every day.

Contents

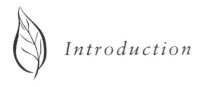

Introduction

YOU'RE PROBABLY READING THIS BOOK BECAUSE YOU OR someone you love has had a miscarriage. Not only have you experienced miscarriage, but the pregnancy you lost came about only because of infertility treatments. You may be realizing that very few people, if anyone, can really understand what you're going through. You might feel angry or guilty, and you can hardly believe that if you want to become pregnant again you'll have to start all over with the medications, the waiting, the ultrasounds and blood tests, and the agony of buying yet another home pregnancy test. It doesn't seem fair. Some women can become pregnant so easily, and some don't even want their pregnancies. But you wanted yours very much, and it was taken away.

Miscarriage can be devastating for any woman. For those who became pregnant through treatment for infertility, miscarriage brings an added layer of frustration and anxiety. As one thirty-nine-year-old woman says, "We'd been through so much already, so much disappointment, so much crying and pain just to become pregnant. Then the miscarriage. It was the most heart-wrenching experience I've ever been through. But the most frustrating part for me is that we can't be like normal couples who can just

go to bed one night and start to conceive another baby.
Why them and not us? I might never get pregnant again."

WHY WRITE THIS BOOK?

We've written this book because we saw a need. One
of the authors, Carrie, persevered through two years of
infertility treatments before becoming pregnant, only to
lose the pregnancy. She searched for books about miscarriage, but none of them addressed her particular situation.
They all suggested the same thing: get pregnant again. Not
such great advice for someone who needed monthly injections to become pregnant just once. She needed a book that
specifically addressed miscarriage after infertility—a book
that would help her understand why it happened, what
other women feel about it, and how she could start to heal.

We hope that this book will serve as a source of vali-
dation and hope for women who, like Carrie, have had a
miscarriage after being treated for infertility. Recovery from
miscarriage is a process that takes time and support from
those you love. Everyone's experience is different, but many
women in this position have some basic feelings in common. They have all struggled to attain something that most
people take for granted—getting pregnant—and when they
have a miscarriage, they realize that they have to deal with
it in a different way than other couples do. Deciding how

to proceed with plans for another pregnancy is a major part of the process.

In preparing to write this book, we spoke to a number of women who miscarried after infertility treatment. They generously shared their stories with us, and their words are woven throughout the book. Carrie also shares her personal account of miscarriage, in chapter 1. Chapter 2 discusses the medical aspects of miscarriage, while chapters 3 through 11 explore the common themes that emerged in our discussions with the women we interviewed. Throughout the book, we offer strategies and suggestions for coping with difficult feelings and coming to terms with what happened.

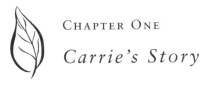

CHAPTER ONE

Carrie's Story

I'LL NEVER FORGET THE DAY OF MY PREGNANCY TEST. My husband, Dave, and I drove all the way to our reproductive endocrinologist's office, sixty miles from our home. We were beside ourselves with anticipation. A few hours later, my doctor called and told me I was pregnant. Unbelievable! The doctor said we should be "cautiously optimistic," but I truly believed that after such a long road we had paid our dues and nothing bad could happen to this pregnancy. I was about to learn that life is not fair.

Dave and I had been married for three years. After trying unsuccessfully for a year to get pregnant, we decided to seek medical help. A few years earlier, I had been diagnosed with polycystic ovary syndrome (PCOS). In this condition, the ovaries are covered with cysts, and ovulation is irregular. We knew that the PCOS would make it more difficult for us to conceive, but we also knew that my older sister had the same condition, and she got pregnant with a few cycles of Clomid. My gynecologist put me on Clomid for a few months, but it didn't work for me. I then sought help from a specialist, a reproductive endocrinologist who was also an expert in PCOS. She began treating me with Repronex, an injectable fertility drug.

I had to have Repronex shots every night for approximately two weeks each month. At first I thought they were painful, and I was afraid of them, but after the first cycle I found I no longer feared needles. The drug seemed to make my mood swings more extreme, but that could have just been the stress of infertility. The first two weeks of the month also included ultrasounds every other day to monitor follicle growth. When the follicle was deemed big enough, I was given an HCG (human chorionic gonadotropin) shot to trigger the follicle's release from the ovary. Then it was time for the IUI, or intrauterine insemination, in which Dave's sperm was "processed" and inserted into my vagina by the doctor. Dave and I were so excited, so full of hope that this could be our month. After the IUI, we had to wait two long weeks to find out if the procedure was successful. And this time, it was!

Six weeks after the positive pregnancy test, on a Friday in November, I was at my office. When I went to the bathroom at 1:00 P.M., I saw a dark brown discharge on the toilet paper. I quickly called my mom, who is a nurse and researcher. She asked me if I had any cramping or saw blood. Since I didn't, she wasn't alarmed. At about five that evening, the discharge was there again. That night I had dinner with a friend, who told me that dark brown spotting was no big deal—when she was twelve weeks pregnant, she had had bleeding, and everything was fine. That made me feel better.

After dinner, I saw a few drops of gooey discharge in the toilet bowl. I was really starting to feel nervous. I looked up "bleeding in early pregnancy" in my pregnancy book. I had no red blood and no cramps, so I relaxed a bit. When I woke up the next morning, however, I expelled a large amount of bloody material into the toilet. I started screaming, shaking, and crying. Deep down, I knew what had just happened. Dave came running into the bathroom; he knew too. We both wanted so much to believe that this was somehow normal, but we knew it wasn't.

I composed myself enough to call work and tell them what I thought might be happening. I actually thought I'd be able to pull myself together to go to work. Later I realized that I was trying desperately to cling to "normalcy." I couldn't be having a miscarriage if I had to go to work, could I? Next I called my mom, and when I told her what had happened, she said, "I'm coming right over." That's when I knew for certain that the pregnancy was over.

After I hung up, I lay on the bed with Dave and waited. I remember kicking my feet and shaking my arms, almost like I was trying to wriggle out of my own skin. My parents arrived a few minutes later. My dad hugged me in the hallway and started to cry—which almost broke my heart. Seeing my parents so sad for me was just awful. A call to my doctor's office confirmed our fears. She said it sounded like a miscarriage, and that we should come right in. I tried to hold on to some tiny scrap of hope that everything was fine.

The doctor was very nice and very gentle, but the ultrasound confirmed that nothing was there anymore, just blood waiting to be expelled. We had the official word — we had lost our baby.

Dave and I cried for hours. It was complete devastation. I kept thinking how unfair it was. We had already been through so much just to get to this point — why did this have to happen? Somewhere inside I believed that because it took so long to get pregnant, we were somehow immune to any further problems.

That first day we stayed on the couch under a big blanket all day, crying, trying to cope, voicing our fears. What if it took another year or more to get pregnant again? What if we couldn't get pregnant again? And if we were lucky enough to become pregnant, what if we had another miscarriage? How could we handle that? We had never even considered the possibility of a miscarriage before it happened to us.

The first few days after the miscarriage seemed to last a year. I told one of my friends that we had lost the baby and asked her to call all my girlfriends. I couldn't bear the thought of going through the story so many times. On Sunday night, I became terribly upset because the weekend was over and I'd have to go back to work, back to a "normal" routine. It was irrational, I knew, but I thought that if I could just stay on the couch, I'd be okay. But life was going to continue, even though it didn't seem possible that it would ever feel normal again.

I went back to work, but I was exhausted. I had a hard time getting up once I was sitting down. Everything I did took twice as much energy. Even the thought of getting off the couch at night to get into bed was too much for me.

For several weeks, strange small things made me cry. When a colleague suggested going to a Japanese restaurant, I burst into tears. I had eaten Japanese food the night before the miscarriage. The one thing that was good during this time was Dave. He was so supportive, listening to me say the same things over and over again, letting me cry, and giving me hugs. At least I wasn't alone. We saw this as "our" problem. I was worried about him, though, because I wasn't sure he was really dealing with the loss. He seemed to be trying to be strong for me. Was that helping him?

Two weeks after the miscarriage was Thanksgiving. The word itself seemed like a bad joke. My mom told me to stay home in my pajamas if I wanted to. I managed to go to dinner at her house, wearing sweatpants and a sweatshirt. I tried to be happy, but I wasn't. Dave put on a brave face.

As we slowly got back to our routines, the big question was what to do about resuming infertility treatments. Should we start right away after my first period? I guess we hadn't given up the fantasy of getting pregnant on our own, because we decided to wait a few months before starting treatment again. We wanted to see if we could conceive without the drugs. Our doctor said that if it was going to happen, it would probably happen in the first two months. If we weren't pregnant by then, she recommended that I start taking Repronex again.

While thinking about a new pregnancy, I was still obsessed with my lost pregnancy. Why had I miscarried? I read more about PCOS and learned that the miscarriage rate could be as high as 45 percent for people with the condition, a frightening statistic. My doctor did say, however, that it was a good sign that my pregnancy had lasted six weeks, and that we should be encouraged for the future. At least this time we were going into the process with our eyes wide open.

I thought that by a month after the miscarriage, I'd be back to my old self, but I still felt bad. The problems we were having with our insurance company didn't help. I found myself crying every time I had to call them, as it required me to actively think about the miscarriage again. That would lead to a cascade of thoughts about how far along I would have been if I hadn't miscarried, how I would have been buying maternity clothes and deciding on baby names.

My first period after the miscarriage was due soon. Could it be possible by some miracle that I wouldn't get a period? That I'd be pregnant with no treatments? I knew the chances were slim, but I couldn't help thinking about it. It made me so angry that most couples just have sex and get pregnant. They have to worry about not getting pregnant instead of getting pregnant. What did we ever do wrong to be faced with this? That night I had some brown spotting, meaning I'd probably get my period the next day. Oh no, I thought, here we go again. I'm not pregnant.

I was reading everything I could about miscarriage. I found it helpful to read about other people's experiences. It bothered me, though, that none of the women in the books had miscarried after conceiving through infertility treatments. Some books suggested that looking forward to another pregnancy could help you resolve your feelings about the miscarriage. But I knew I might never have another pregnancy.

Although I wanted to get beyond the miscarriage, thinking about it was a way to reassure myself that I really had been pregnant. One book had some ideas about how to honor and remember the lost baby. Following the book's advice, I bought a little ring with rubies, which would have been my baby's birthstone. The ring helped me feel connected to the experience.

By Christmas I was feeling a little better. Dave and I had had several talks about the miscarriage, and he had cried a few more times, so I was less concerned that he was burying his feelings to help me. My mom suggested that I might be able to sort out my feelings by writing about my experiences in a journal. Perhaps the journal could lead to a research project or a book. It comforted me to think that I might be able to help other women in my situation.

Dave worried that by working on the journal I would cause more pain for myself, but when I started writing I found that it did help me. He soon saw that the project was helping me to focus on something bigger than my personal experience.

Just when things seemed to be getting a little easier and I wasn't thinking about the miscarriage all the time, I was confronted by a challenge. At our friends' annual holiday party, I finally had to see my friend who was pregnant. My other girlfriends all made a big fuss over her. I understood that, and knew it was natural, but I still felt overwhelmed. I hid in the bathroom so they wouldn't see me crying. My friend deserved the attention. I was really happy for her, but I couldn't stop crying. I even started to hyperventilate.

One of my friends came in the bathroom. She hugged me, let me have a good cry, and listened to me talk. I was supposed to be pregnant too! Everyone should have been fussing over both of us, rubbing both our bellies. I was so ashamed, but I couldn't help my feelings. That was a tough day.

A few months later, two of my friends gave birth. For the first time since my miscarriage, I found myself in a baby store, buying gifts for them. I remembered that they had both started trying to conceive a year after I did. They both had baby girls, which is what I had wanted. I suddenly was consumed with sadness, feeling completely hopeless that we'd ever have a baby. Then I started worrying about what would happen if I did get pregnant. Could I sustain the pregnancy? No one knew why I miscarried the first time. What was to keep it from happening again?

In February, I reluctantly admitted that my hopes for ovulating without medication were just a fantasy, and we decided to go back to infertility treatments. Unfortunately, that also meant going back to the hassles of dealing with the insurance company. I was determined, however, to keep a positive attitude about this cycle. It would work. I had to believe that.

This time around, having the injections didn't seem like such a big deal. But after the insemination, I started to cry as soon as the nurse left the room. I felt so vulnerable! The situation was totally out of my control. It always was, I knew, but once the IUI was done, there was nothing to do but wait. At least when we were administering the shots, we were actively doing something to get pregnant. The waiting was harder this time than it had been before. I found myself analyzing every possible symptom, telling myself that I probably wasn't pregnant. I knew that my sore breasts were likely due to the HCG shot, not a pregnancy. Every time I went to the bathroom, I expected to see red on the toilet paper.

Two weeks later when I got my period, I felt disgusted at the failure of another treatment cycle. Everyone said that my attitude could make a difference, but how could I stay optimistic when everything was always negative? How could I keep thinking positive thoughts when all I got was bad news? A few people started talking to me about adoption, but Dave and I just weren't ready to think about that. Maybe later, but not then.

So we started another cycle of Repronex. If we didn't keep trying, we figured, it would never happen. My sister said it was exciting—we had a clean slate and could possibly be pregnant in just a few weeks. I tried to adopt her positive outlook, but without much success. Every cycle cost us about $600, not to mention the long trips to the fertility clinic and all the shots I had to endure. How many more times could we do this?

People started telling me stories about a cousin (friend, aunt, neighbor) who tried for years and years to get pregnant, and just as the couple gave up, boom, she got pregnant. I quickly got sick of those stories. Was the point supposed to be that I'd also have to endure many years of fertility treatments and go into debt, only to get pregnant as soon as I filled out the adoption papers? Was this supposed to comfort me? It didn't. I knew that people meant well, but I wished they would just say they were sorry for what Dave and I were going through or that they were thinking of us.

I can't even describe how upset I was when I got my period after our third IUI since the miscarriage. Not only was I not pregnant, but Dave had recently found out that he had to go away for business for four months (coming home just on weekends). This cycle had been our last chance before Dave's trip. I was obsessed with getting pregnant, and I hated the idea of waiting four months to start treatments again.

I was also concerned about why the IUIs weren't working. If the doctor determined that insemination was not helping us, the next step would be in vitro fertilization (IVF). We'd have to spend our entire savings just to do one cycle of IVF. And there were no guarantees with that either. I felt I couldn't possibly handle having a miscarriage after spending $10,000 to get pregnant. Sometimes I thought I was going crazy.

I just couldn't wait to do the next IUI. I told Dave that I wanted to go ahead with the next cycle, which would be in a week or two. I could get my mom to give me my shots, and I could drive to the doctor's office by myself. The only tricky part would be getting Dave home on the day of the IUI. I begged him to tell his boss that he would need to fly home for one day—and then he could go right back. After a lengthy discussion, Dave agreed to talk to his boss.

As it turned out, Dave was home when the IUI needed to be done, which we took as a good sign. And even though my insurance company had decided not to pay for this IUI, I felt good about it. My positive attitude was finally kicking in. Fourteen days after the IUI, I had not gotten my period, so Dave and I drove up to the clinic for a blood pregnancy test. I was trying to keep my expectations low, but I was very hopeful.

When the phone rang that afternoon, I nervously picked it up. My doctor said, "Carrie, you're pregnant!" I screamed and asked her if she was lying. She assured me she wasn't and told me to come back in two days for another blood test to be sure that my HCG levels were rising. Dave and I couldn't calm down. Could it be? Had it really worked? It took about fifteen minutes before we looked at each other and realized that this might not last. We couldn't feel completely joyful about the news. As the days went on, I became more and more scared about losing the baby.

I was pregnant, but things were not the way I thought they would be. Even a few months into the pregnancy, I was convinced that it was just a matter of time before I lost this baby too. Every time I went to the bathroom, I looked for blood, wondering when it was coming. Intellectually I knew this was not a good way to behave, but I couldn't help it. Seeing the early ultrasound pictures didn't help. I was a mess, just waiting for the other shoe to drop. I found myself crying for no real reason. I started looking forward to the twenty-week point, because I figured that if I lost the baby then, it would be considered a stillbirth, and people would take a stillbirth more seriously than a miscarriage.

My mom and sister were concerned about me and suggested that I see a therapist. Although I felt kind of defensive about it, I realized that ever since the miscarriage, I had been different. After struggling for so long to become pregnant, this should have been a happy time. Yet I was miserable. I was constantly on edge and annoyed with everyone.

Going to a therapist was the best thing I could have done. She helped me understand my anger and grief about the miscarriage, as well as my fears about the new pregnancy. I began to manage my stress much better and relax and enjoy my pregnancy more. I found out that I was carrying a girl, and knowing the gender also helped put my mind at ease. Sometimes I still couldn't believe that I was pregnant, but I slowly became less fearful that something would go wrong. Some people say that when you struggle to get pregnant, then you enjoy it much more. For me, it took a long time to stop being afraid that I would lose the pregnancy. Eventually, I did give birth to a healthy baby.

My heart aches for all the women who have had a miscarriage and are being treated for infertility. It's a hard journey—I know how hard it is. I hope this book helps you, if even a little.

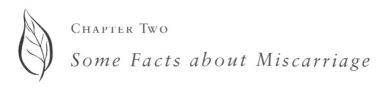

CHAPTER TWO

Some Facts about Miscarriage

YOU MAY BE SURPRISED TO LEARN THAT NO GOVERNMENT agencies or professional organizations collect data about how many women have miscarriages in the United States. Therefore, the true incidence of miscarriage is not known. Many women who miscarry don't go to a doctor because they didn't realize they were pregnant. When women do seek medical attention for miscarriage, doctors are not required to report it the way they have to record a birth or death.

So how frequent is miscarriage? Some researchers estimate that between 12 percent and 31 percent of all conceptions end in miscarriage in the first or second trimester. Other scientists believe that the early pregnancy loss rate is actually closer to 50 percent because of the high number of unrecognized miscarriages that occur as early as two to four weeks after conception. Based on these estimates, a reasonable guess is that perhaps one-third to one-half of all pregnancies end in miscarriage.

Many people are surprised to learn these statistics. Miscarriage is much more common than most people realize. Even in an information-soaked world, most people don't hear much about miscarriage. While many formerly hidden subjects, such as sexuality, cancer, menopause, and rape, are now discussed openly, miscarriage seems to be an exception. Perhaps the pain of miscarriage is just too deep. Perhaps women don't know how many others have suffered the same loss.

Miscarriage occurs for many different reasons. About 80 percent of miscarriages happen during the first trimester, and researchers believe that many of these are due to chromosome problems in the fetus. Most women who have a miscarriage in the first trimester of pregnancy never find out why it happened.

TYPES OF MISCARRIAGE

When physicians talk about miscarriage, they sometimes use the term "spontaneous abortion." This wording can be upsetting, since to the general public the word "abortion" usually means a pregnancy that is terminated intentionally. But doctors call any pregnancy loss before twenty weeks of gestation an abortion. In medical terminology, an elective abortion is the termination of a pregnancy by choice. A spontaneous abortion is an unplanned pregnancy loss—in other words, a miscarriage. Many healthcare providers try not to use the word "abortion" when talking to a woman who has suffered a miscarriage, because the word carries such a heavy emotional burden. If your provider does say "spontaneous abortion" when discussing your miscarriage, he or she is not being thoughtless, but just using precise medical terminology.

Not all miscarriages are alike. The later in pregnancy a miscarriage occurs, the more symptoms a woman usually experiences. Miscarriage before the sixth week of pregnancy might be experienced as a heavy period; miscarriage between seven and twelve weeks might be more uncomfortable and include more bleeding and cramping. Miscarriages after thirteen weeks can feel like real labor.

There are several types of miscarriage, each with a different medical name. Your provider might use one of these terms in your medical record to describe what he or she finds when examining you.

Threatened miscarriage

In threatened miscarriage (or abortion), the pregnancy is still intact but may not be able to be maintained. Symptoms include spotting (not heavy vaginal bleeding) and mild uterine cramps. No pregnancy tissue has passed through the vagina, and the cervix is closed. If you're diagnosed with threatened miscarriage, it doesn't mean that you will definitely miscarry, but your provider will be concerned. You will likely be advised to stay in bed and avoid any sexual activity.

Inevitable miscarriage

With this diagnosis, there's a moderate amount of bleeding, with mild to severe cramping. Although no pregnancy tissue has passed from the vagina, the cervix is dilated. Cervical dilation, accompanied by the other symptoms, indicates that the miscarriage is going to occur imminently. There's probably no chance of maintaining the pregnancy. Within a number of hours, the pregnancy tissue is likely to pass out of the vagina.

Incomplete miscarriage

This term refers to a miscarriage in which some, but not all, of the pregnancy tissue has been expelled. Symptoms include heavy bleeding, severe cramping, and dilation of the cervix. If you have an incomplete miscarriage, you may need to have a D & C (dilation and curettage). In this procedure, your cervix is dilated (widened) and the inside of your uterus is scraped to remove all pregnancy tissue ("curettage" means scraping). Having the D & C is important because if any pregnancy tissue remains in your uterus, you can continue to bleed, which can lead to infection or other serious problems.

Complete miscarriage

If your provider diagnoses a complete miscarriage, it means that the pregnancy tissue has already been expelled. At this point, there is only slight bleeding and mild cramping, and the cervix is no longer dilated. You already had cramping, bleeding, and dilation of the cervix along with the expulsion of the pregnancy contents. If complete miscarriage is diagnosed, you will probably not need a D & C. The worst physical symptoms are over.

Missed abortion (miscarriage)

This term means that the fetus has died, but no actual miscarriage has occurred. This can be a particularly difficult diagnosis for a woman and her family, because no real symptoms of miscarriage are present, yet the pregnancy has ended. There is no bleeding or cramping and no cervical dilation. The pregnancy loss may be discovered during a prenatal office visit when a fetal heartbeat isn't heard, or during an ultrasound examination when the provider sees that the fetus is no longer moving. Sometimes a woman's uterus is not getting larger, as expected during pregnancy. With this type of miscarriage, it is essential to do a D & C to remove the pregnancy tissue.

Septic miscarriage

In this uncommon condition, an incomplete miscarriage becomes infected (septic). Symptoms include fever, cramping, and a foul-smelling vaginal discharge. Women who have a septic miscarriage need to have a D & C and prompt treatment with antibiotics.

Recurrent miscarriage

Women who are diagnosed with recurrent miscarriage (also called habitual miscarriage) have had three or more miscarriages. Several treatments are available, depending on the cause of the problem, but none are guaranteed to work. One option is "cerclage," a surgical procedure to sew the cervix shut to help prevent miscarriages. Cerclage doesn't work for all women who have recurrent miscarriages, however. Sometimes recurrent miscarriage is caused by genetic problems, and your provider might suggest genetic counseling. Some women never find out the cause.

Ectopic pregnancy

Although not technically a miscarriage, an ectopic pregnancy ends in the loss of a pregnancy. In an ectopic pregnancy, the fertilized egg implants somewhere other than the uterus, most commonly in a fallopian tube. Rarely, the egg may implant in the cervix, an ovary, or the abdominal organs. The uterus is the only place designed to maintain and nurture a pregnancy. Normally, about six to ten days after fertilization, the zygote, or fertilized egg, travels down the fallopian tube into the uterus, where it implants firmly and grows for the next nine months. Sometimes, for reasons not fully understood, the zygote implants in the tiny fallopian tube instead. As the zygote expands, the woman starts to experience abdominal pain. If the problem is not discovered, the fallopian tube can rupture, causing bleeding, pain, and even death. Ectopic pregnancy can be damaging to a woman's future fertility.

Fortunately, most ectopic pregnancies are diagnosed well before a woman has any symptoms. Ultrasound (images, also called "sonograms," made from sound) early in pregnancy can show whether the fertilized egg has implanted in the uterus or the fallopian tube. The usual

D & C

To remove the remains of the pregnancy from your uterus after a miscarriage, your doctor may do a dilation and curettage (also called a D & C). Typically you'll be admitted to the hospital, but you probably won't have to stay overnight. The procedure itself generally takes less than an hour.

At the hospital, you're given anesthesia. Although the doctor doesn't have to cut anything, the scraping of the uterus would hurt too much without the anesthesia. During the procedure, you're in the same position as for a regular vaginal examination (legs in stirrups). Most women don't feel much pain afterward. You might have some cramps and light bleeding. Your doctor will want you to take it easy for a few days when you go home.

treatment for ectopic pregnancy is surgery to remove the pregnancy tissue. Often the tube is removed as well, because it's difficult to remove the zygote without destroying the tube. Some doctors use medications to help expel the pregnancy without surgery, but not all women are candidates for these medicines.

MISCARRIAGE AND INFERTILITY

You've probably read a lot about infertility, especially if you've received treatment for it. In the United States, about five million people of reproductive age suffer from infertility. It is diagnosed after a year or more of unprotected sexual intercourse during ovulation (or timed for ovulation) without a pregnancy.

Most people who are unable to conceive a child wonder what's causing the problem. They may blame themselves or their partner. Research has shown that women and men are about equally likely to be infertile. Approximately 35 percent of the time, infertility occurs because of a problem in the woman's body, and about 35 percent of the time it stems from a problem in the man's body. About 20 percent of the time, infertility results from combined problems in the couple, and about 10 percent of the time, the cause cannot be found. If infertility is suspected, both members of the couple need to be evaluated.

There are many possible causes of infertility. Some women don't ovulate, or don't ovulate often enough. A woman's fallopian tubes may be closed, or she may have scar tissue or other problems inside the uterus. Women who are over forty may have stopped ovulating or may ovulate less frequently, making it difficult to conceive. Some women have had their reproductive organs removed because of cancer or another disease. In men, a structural problem can block the flow of sperm or cause low sperm counts. Some men have had cancer or an infection that affected their reproductive organs. Some men have problems with their hormone levels, which affects their sperm quality.

Treatment for infertility depends on the cause. Treatment may involve surgery, oral medications, injectable

SYMPTOMS OF MISCARRIAGE

Symptoms of miscarriage include vaginal bleeding or spotting and uterine cramping. The bleeding may look like dark-colored mucus or red blood. Depending on how far along the pregnancy is, the fetus may be expelled. The discharge might look like clots or gooey tissue. It might continue to come out over a few hours, a bit at a time.

A miscarriage can also take place without producing any symptoms. It may be discovered when a doctor or nurse observes that the fetal heartbeat is missing, your abdomen is not growing, or an infection has started in the uterus.

If you think you might be miscarrying, contact your doctor promptly. Tell the provider exactly what symptoms you are having, how much bleeding is occurring, and if you have expelled anything other than blood from your vagina. Describe the color and consistency of any vaginal discharge. If you develop a fever, call your provider immediately. You may have an infection, which could be life threatening.

Not much can be done to prevent a miscarriage once it has begun, but it is essential that the contents of the uterus be expelled to prevent infection and hemorrhage. This may require hospitalization and a dilation and curettage (D & C) procedure.

medications, in vitro fertilization (IVF), or other techniques for helping a pregnancy get started. Some treatments use the couple's own sperm and eggs, while others rely on donor sperm or donor eggs.

The incidence of miscarriage is not necessarily higher among women who've become pregnant after being treated for infertility than it is for women without the complication of infertility. While infertility itself doesn't place a woman at greater risk for miscarriage, women undergoing infertility treatments often have other risk factors. For example, women over age thirty-five have twice the risk of miscarriage as younger women. For women over age forty-five, the chance of miscarrying is 50 percent. Women who have had three or more pregnancy losses also face a higher risk. Many women being treated for infertility are over thirty-five, and they may have had multiple pregnancy losses. They are therefore at higher risk for miscarriage than the average woman.

THE PSYCHOLOGICAL EFFECTS OF INFERTILITY AND MISCARRIAGE

Studies of women who are diagnosed as infertile and who participate in infertility treatment reveal feelings of stigmatization and high levels of depression. One study found high levels of anxiety and agitation in women undergoing in vitro fertilization. Another describes infertility as a life crisis and suggests that women who plan to begin infertility treatments require intervention to help them move through the continuum of grief and resolve their feelings.

Almost all studies of the psychological effects of miscarriage have involved women with normal fertility. These studies suggest that miscarriage, like infertility, is a life-changing event. Women who've had a miscarriage commonly experience feelings of emptiness, dread, guilt, and grief. They have an increased need for support, and they express fears about their future childbearing ability. Many women have higher levels of depression and anxiety for up to a year after a miscarriage. Posttraumatic stress disorder has also been reported after miscarriage.

Research shows that women who have experienced miscarriage look to a future pregnancy as a primary method for resolving grief, although they might still fear the loss of subsequent pregnancies. One study found that women who do not conceive or give birth by one year after their miscarriage have a higher risk for depressive symptoms. Women are also more likely to experience intense and long-lasting distress following miscarriage if they strongly desired the pregnancy, waited a long time to conceive, or have no living children. These factors typically apply to women who miscarry after infertility treatment.

Since future pregnancy is a large factor in healing the grief felt by fertile women who have had a miscarriage, how does pregnancy loss affect women whose future fertility is far from assured? What do these women feel? The following chapters describe some of those feelings and what women have done to cope.

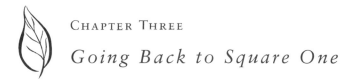

CHAPTER THREE

Going Back to Square One

MANY WOMEN DESCRIBE INFERTILITY AS AN EMOTIONAL roller coaster and say that having a miscarriage after infertility treatment only adds to that feeling. Infertile couples face despair about their inability to conceive, uncertainty and anxiety about whether treatments will work, and renewed grief each month that a pregnancy does not occur. When a pregnancy test is finally positive, some women are elated while others are guardedly optimistic. For some women, the thought of miscarrying never occurs; others fear it so much that they find it hard to fully embrace the pregnancy. For both groups, however, miscarriage leads to deeper despair.

Women who miscarry after infertility treatments feel they have already "been through so much just to get pregnant," and now they have to go "back to square one." Going back to square one means going back to not being pregnant and going back to infertility. It often involves launching another series of treatments, figuring out how to pay for treatment, and coping with feelings such as grief and anger.

"We'd been dealing with infertility for four years before I finally became pregnant," one woman recalls.

"Along with being disappointed about the miscarriage, I felt total disbelief. I couldn't believe this happened after everything we'd been through. I remember feeling that if I could take my skin off my body and just melt, I'd feel a lot better." Another woman says, "Treatments again? I don't know. I'm just trying to make myself excited about trying again."

BACK TO FINANCIAL BURDENS

Couples who resume infertility treatment take on additional financial burdens as well. Many couples have no insurance for infertility treatment, and those who do have coverage know that it won't last indefinitely. As one woman comments, "Because of the financial commitment, the urgency for success is magnified." For another woman, the loss of her pregnancy also represented a real loss of money: "That was a big hurdle to get over—doing all this financially, taking a risk, and then losing all that money."

Other women express concern about having to pay for infertility treatments long after the miscarriage. "I knew the infertility treatments were costly and not guaranteed, but I didn't really believe I'd have to start again." "We've spent so much money already. And who's got the money to keep doing it? You get pregnant and you lose it, but you still have to pay everything off for two or three years

RESOLVING FINANCIAL ISSUES

For couples dealing with infertility, financial issues can be a major source of anxiety. A miscarriage represents a great deal of lost money for couples who needed infertility treatments to become pregnant. But the immediate period following the miscarriage is not the time to try to resolve financial issues with the hospital or your insurance company. Wait a few weeks, until your head is clearer and you can think better, to discuss your financial situation and find realistic ways to handle this financial burden.

after." "At least my insurance paid for some of it, but I still owed $1,200 from the last treatments, and at that point I didn't even have a pregnancy. It took me months to pay that off before we could try again."

One woman sums up the financial aspect of her experience as "a cruel joke." "I thought it was over, finally. No more big payments—you're finally pregnant. And then you miscarry. Sometimes it makes me mad that this whole thing is a big moneymaking business as much as anything else."

BACK TO DESPAIR AND ANGER

For many women who miscarry, starting a new series of infertility treatments brings up a mixture of despair and anger. One woman remembers, "I realized that having more treatments meant I had to keep this job. I don't really like it. I have to work a job where I can be off half a day to do treatments. It's hard to find a place that lets you do that."

Another woman says that even though she is afraid of having more treatments, she isn't ready to give up: "It's such a good feeling to be pregnant. I want that feeling again. Really, you never want to give up trying." Some women begin to explore other options: "We're looking into adoption, too, but there's a part of me holding back from making those commitments, because I'm not ready to let go of getting pregnant."

CHAPTER FOUR

A *Struggle between Hope and Hopelessness*

INITIATING INFERTILITY TREATMENTS IS A HOPEFUL ACT. You're doing something proactive to become pregnant, and you hope that it will work. You have hopes for the pregnancy and for the child you may have. When a pregnancy occurs after infertility treatments, hope is often magnified, but it can be troublesome. If you have lost pregnancies in the past, you might be afraid to allow yourself to think that this one will last. Or perhaps you decide that your pregnancy woes are behind you, and you bond to the pregnancy, choose a name for your child, and tell all your relatives. Then the bleeding or the cramps start, and your hopefulness disappears along with the pregnancy.

Most people feel helpless at times after a miscarriage. How can you find the will to go on and consider future parenthood? This is a fundamental question for women who experience miscarriage after infertility.

THE DIFFICULTY OF REMAINING HOPEFUL

All the women we interviewed expressed the difficulty of remaining hopeful after a miscarriage. They have felt hopeless and helpless about their own fertility. "This leaves me hopeless again," says one woman. "I try to make myself excited about trying again, but I can't. Just becoming pregnant was such a major accomplishment for me, but will that be all I have?"

Despite their despair, women try to reassure themselves that they have not reached the end of possible treatments for their infertility, and that perhaps the next time they will conceive and retain a healthy pregnancy. "I just know I will have a baby someday," says one woman. "I have to believe that."

Some women who feel hopeless about their fertility begin considering adoption. The thought that they can adopt gives them hope for becoming a parent someday, but at the same time they don't want to give up hope of having a successful pregnancy. Most women say they would consider adoption only when all other options have failed. For these women, adoption is an admission of defeat: "I can't adopt. Adoption is for when all hope is gone."

LINGERING HOPELESSNESS

The struggle between being hopeful and losing all hope is common among women who experience miscarriage after infertility. Despite their best efforts to remain hopeful, many women say they still fall into hopelessness: "Miscarriage for me could mean no children ever." "I'm just not sure I want to go through it all over again. Start a new

GRIEVING AFTER MISCARRIAGE

After a miscarriage, it's common to feel overwhelming sadness, despair, or anguish. It's often best to let these feelings of grief wash over you. Cry as often as you need to. Stay in bed for a few days, or hibernate on the couch. Talk to only the people you want to talk to. If you chose to tell family and friends about the pregnancy, you probably have many who share your grief. Take advantage of that, and allow them to care for you.

It may take days or weeks to get over the first phase of sadness after losing a pregnancy. For some women it takes longer. Grieving is an individual experience, and everyone feels it differently. Generally, however, if a week has passed since the miscarriage and you're having trouble functioning—you can't get out of bed or can't get yourself to work—it might be a good idea to find some help. Perhaps your healthcare provider or a good friend can give you the name of a reputable counselor or therapist.

procedure and go through all that. It's very painful, and I don't know if it's in God's plan for me. I'm kind of in a holding pattern." "It seems like if you don't have infertility issues, chances are you're going to have another pregnancy. Whereas for people like me who are dealing with infertility, and who didn't get pregnant on their own, and who have had a miscarriage, the odds of getting pregnant again are a lot lower, a lot slimmer, so I think our outlook is a lot more bleak."

COPING WITH HOPELESSNESS

Feelings of hopelessness are normal during the intense grieving after a miscarriage. Most couples ultimately find a way to live with alternating feelings of hopelessness and hopefulness. Trying to keep a positive attitude most of the time is best for your mental health, but don't beat yourself up if you give in to hopelessness at times. If it seems like those feelings are starting to take over your life, however, you may need professional help to resolve them.

The first few weeks after a miscarriage are probably the worst time to think about your future fertility, but such thoughts are difficult to avoid. Remember that you have been hopeful in the past, and hope will return to your life—it's just going to take some time.

When the time comes to make a decision about whether to resume infertility treatments, you will probably struggle again with hope versus hopelessness. Be ready for that, and if the bad feelings do not fade, seek a counselor who can help you with your grief.

Chapter Five

Running Out of Time

Most women involved with infertility treatment worry about the biological clock. It is common for women to seek treatment after age thirty-five, when fertility starts to decline, even among women with no reproductive problems. Women in their mid- to late thirties realize that they don't have many years in which to become pregnant, especially if they want more than one child. If miscarriage occurs after a much-desired pregnancy, the time crunch becomes even more acute.

Women who have miscarried after infertility treatment say they feel time pressure. Many realize that because of their age they do not have many years left before menopause. Others worry that their bodies can't take much more of the medications used to induce ovulation. Some women feel that their families have had enough of the constant struggle for pregnancy, and that it has taken too long already. "I'm putting my family through so much," one woman notes. "How much longer can we try? How much more can my body take?"

The infertility process can make couples obsess about time, keeping track of the days for injections, going to a string of ultrasound appointments, charting cycle days, being available for IUIs, and waiting the interminable two weeks for a pregnancy test. For these couples, time becomes an oppressive cloud over their heads. A miscarriage only worsens the pressure. Should they start treatments again, and when? Should they take any time off? If so, how much?

LIFE IN THE FUTURE

The need to quickly become pregnant again is not the only time pressure women feel after miscarriage. They express concerns about what the rest of their life will hold for them: "It's hard to think that you're going to grow old and never have children. I grew up in a big family, and to make a family it takes more than a husband and wife. That's how I always felt. My husband and I really aren't a family because there are no children. It took a long time to get over that." "I never thought I'd be here. My age and can't have children? This isn't what my life was going to be."

EMPLOYMENT AND FINANCIAL ISSUES

Women dealing with infertility and miscarriage also feel significant time pressures related to their employment outside the home. "I was pregnant, so I quit my job and everything, and now I'm not pregnant. What do I do?" one woman wonders. Some women say they had to take sick days and vacation days to accommodate their infertility treatments. When they needed more time off after the miscarriage, they worried about their job security. "At least the miscarriage happened while I was on vacation, so I didn't have to take any more time off from work," says one woman.

At the same time, some women wonder whether they should quit their jobs and dedicate themselves to becoming pregnant again. "Maybe the stress of my job made me miscarry," one woman says. "I don't think so, but maybe."

The financial strain of infertility treatments makes these decisions even more difficult. "My boss is good to me and gives me time off, but will that go on forever?" one woman asks. Another worries, "If I leave my job and then I never have a baby, will I get another job this good? Maybe I'm not going to be a mother, and then I'll be working forever."

DEALING WITH TIME CONCERNS

Worries about running out of time are common among women who have had a miscarriage after infertility. It may help to talk to your healthcare provider directly about your concerns. When you're ready to go back to your infertility specialist, tell him or her that you want to talk honestly and realistically about your chances for another conception and about whether and when to begin treatments again.

If you're worried about the time constraints imposed by your job, discuss your concerns with your partner and perhaps with your employer to determine ways to ease the pressure. Perhaps your employer will allow you to work on a reduced schedule for a few months to help you recover from the miscarriage and resume infertility treatments.

Finally, if you're troubled by the thought that you might reach old age without ever having children, try to stop putting your valuable energy into these worries. It's impossible to know how you'll feel when you get older. People's life situations change frequently, and everyone adapts eventually. If you must worry, it's probably more fruitful to think about your current life situation than the future. The steps you take to deal with infertility and miscarriage matter more today, because of how they affect your life right now, than they will tomorrow.

CHAPTER SIX

Anger

ANGER IS PERHAPS THE MOST COMMON EMOTION DESCRIBED by women who miscarry after infertility treatments. Many women don't quite know who they're angry with or how to channel their feelings. One woman comments, "I've been really mad. But who am I angry at? Myself? My body?" Some express anger toward their healthcare providers, God, their families, or couples who seem to take pregnancy for granted. Some women are simply angry about what happened.

ANGER WITH FAMILY

While family can be very supportive, some women find themselves angry at family members who are not helpful. As one woman explains, "I've been angry with my own mother because she didn't even want me to do in vitro. She felt I was taking it out of God's hands, that if it was meant to be it would happen. I completely disagree. I think God gave man knowledge to do these things, and that's the way I look at it. I wouldn't let her stop me from doing it. Now that I've miscarried, everyone expects me to get over it right away—like you can just get over it."

ANGER WITH PREGNANT FRIENDS

Many women say that one of the hardest parts of their experience was being surrounded by friends and family members who had babies or were pregnant. These women often had to take a step back from seeing those friends in the weeks following the miscarriage. One woman decided not to attend a friend's baby shower, which was held three weeks after her miscarriage. She felt it would be too painful to see the baby clothes and hear everyone talking about babies. She sent a gift but told her friend she wasn't feeling well enough to go to the shower. Although she feels guilty about the decision, she knows she did the right thing.

Another woman recalls, "It was especially hard because my friend was having a baby any day, so there was this anticipation—how was I going to deal with it? Of course I didn't hate her or anything, but I'm embarrassed to say I was pretty upset when she had her baby."

ANGER ABOUT NOT BEING "NORMAL"

"The most frustrating part for me is that we can't be like normal couples and go to bed one night and start to conceive another baby," says one woman. "That makes me so mad. Why can't we be like other couples? What did they do to be so lucky?"

Women often find it difficult to resolve their feelings about not being able to become pregnant like "normal" couples. Other couples have to worry about preventing pregnancy or becoming pregnant before they're ready. In contrast, many infertile couples are willing to go to great lengths to become pregnant, then they may lose the pregnancy. "People get pregnant every day and they don't even want to be pregnant, or they didn't try," one woman says. "Why do I have to go through this?" Another reflects, "It's always a little bit poignant when I find out someone is pregnant. Why them and not me?"

ANGER WITH PARENTS WHO TREAT THEIR CHILDREN BADLY

Many women find themselves furious with parents who seem abusive to their children. These women say that the unfairness of their situation, coupled with their strong desire for parenthood, fuels their anger. "I'm still trying to figure out how to deal with my anger at people, like women who are mean to their kids. I just want to say, 'Do you know how lucky you are?' It's really aggravating." "You watch the news and hear about people doing things to their children—it's so frustrating. I want to go find them and shake them."

COPING WITH ANGER

Anger is a powerful emotion, and it can be frightening or make you uncomfortable. Everyone handles anger in his or her own way, but most therapists suggest that it's best to deal with it by getting it out. Here are some suggestions for handling anger in constructive ways:

Choose a safe time when you're alone and allow yourself to scream and yell, punch some pillows, and fully feel your rage.

Give yourself a break from other people's pregnancies and babies. If you're still grieving your miscarriage, don't put yourself in situations where you'll have to pretend to be excited about someone else's pregnancy or new baby, such as a baby shower, bris, or christening. You can tell your friends and family you'll make it up to them in the future, but right now you're not doing well. When you feel better, you can visit with those friends and be excited for their happiness.

A trusted clergy member can be a good source of solace if you feel angry with God. Ask a clergyperson whom you feel comfortable with for help in resolving your feelings. Most clergy are trained in grief counseling.

If family members say things that are not appropriate, such as, "You took it out of God's hands, and now look what happened," it's okay to be angry. Tell them that what they're saying isn't helping you to overcome your grief. You may choose to take a break from talking to these people about your experience until you're feeling better. It's fine to decide to talk only with people you know will be supportive.

🌿 Your anger should lessen over time. If you can't resolve your anger on your own, it's important to seek help. If you're still feeling very angry a few weeks to a month after your miscarriage, you may want to talk to a counselor.

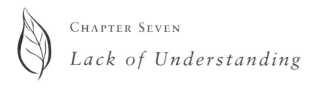

CHAPTER SEVEN

Lack of Understanding

EVEN IF YOU HAVE A LOT OF FRIENDS AND A LARGE FAMILY that loves you, you still may feel that they don't understand what you've been through. This is normal, but it can feel bad. The women we spoke to perceive that no one can really understand what they've experienced. They believe that many people don't understand miscarriage, thinking it's nothing to be concerned about or that the pregnancy wasn't "real." The subject is mysterious to much of the public, since for decades women have been silent about miscarriage and have suffered alone, without talking about it.

Even women who have strong, loving marriages sometimes find that their husbands don't understand. One woman says, "My husband doesn't care if we adopt or have a pregnancy. I don't agree with him. I feel like I need to have something inside me—to feel it grow. I've dreamt about it all my life."

PEOPLE SAYING THE WRONG THING

Many women have been upset by friends and acquaintances saying what one women calls "asinine things." You may have heard statements like these: "At least you know you can get pregnant." "My cousin had lots of miscarriages, and now she has five children." "You can try again." "You'll get over it and forget it ever happened."

One woman remembers, "When I miscarried, people said, 'At least you got pregnant.' That was no help at all." Another says, "Everybody tells me that it's God's will, it was meant to be, and it's God's way of taking care of something that wasn't right. And of course people don't know what to say, but you don't want to hear any of that." A third woman adds, "People say, 'Next time it will be different.' But they don't know. Until you've been in my position, you don't know how it feels. Especially when you know you have a medical problem and it's so hard to get pregnant."

Many people have no idea what to say to a woman who has miscarried after infertility treatments. People don't mean to be thoughtless, but they may say something insensitive or hurtful. "Well, at least you didn't get to know the baby" and "At least it happened early in the pregnancy" are two common reactions that can make you feel worse.

Try to remember that your friends and family don't mean to upset you. Miscarriage is a difficult subject for many people. When someone says something particularly unhelpful, gently tell them that it would be best if they just expressed their sorrow for your situation by saying something like, "I'm so sorry for what happened."

FINDING SUPPORT AND UNDERSTANDING

Women who miscarry after infertility treatments commonly feel that no one can understand what they're going through. In some ways, they are correct. Probably, only others who have had the same experience can truly understand. Make an effort to find those women, perhaps through a support group in your community or online. RESOLVE is one support group offered at many community agencies and hospitals. Call your local hospital to see if they have such a group. Check the resource list on pages 81 to 83 for other organizations that provide support.

If you can't find an appropriate support group in your community, ask your provider if he or she wants to collaborate with you to begin a group. This could be a very therapeutic move on your part.

PEOPLE SAYING NOTHING AT ALL

Equally upsetting is interaction with people who don't even acknowledge the miscarriage. Women say they feel hurt and perceive a lack of understanding when family, friends, and outsiders don't say anything about the miscarriage. One woman recounted a telephone conversation with a relative who knew about her miscarriage but neglected to mention it or say he was sorry.

It's easy to feel that people who don't say anything about your miscarriage don't care about what happened. But this is probably not true. People often find it difficult to broach the topic of grief and loss with women who have miscarried. They might not know what to say or how best to console you, or they may not want to bring it up for fear of making you relive the experience.

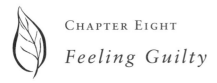

CHAPTER EIGHT

Feeling Guilty

FEW WOMEN EVER FIND OUT WHAT CAUSED THEIR MISCAR-riage, because the majority of miscarriages don't have an identifiable cause. This may be one of the most difficult aspects of the experience. It's easy to obsess about what caused the miscarriage and how it could have been prevented. This can be quite destructive to the recovery process.

Most of the women interviewed for this book were told there was no specific reason for their miscarriage, but they still felt guilty. Although most of them say they know they didn't cause it, they wonder if there was something they could have done to prevent it: "I know in my head that there was nothing I could have done, but trying to get my heart to realize it...." "It makes me wonder. Did I do something wrong?"

It's natural to want to know why things happen. We're trained from the earliest age to examine our mistakes to be sure we don't make the same mistake twice. Women who miscarry want to know why it happened, and "There's no known reason" is not an acceptable answer. That's where the guilt comes in—you may start thinking, "Well, it must have been something I did."

As one woman says, "Not having a reason for the miscarriage makes the experience harder. Did I garden? Pick up something? I have a hard time accepting that it happened for no reason. No one can give me a reason. There must be a reason." Another explains, "I was so afraid it was something I did. Maybe I did something wrong. Maybe it was when I did that load of laundry, or when we had sex."

GUILT ABOUT INFERTILITY

For many women, it's hard to separate feelings of guilt about the miscarriage from the guilt they feel about their infertility. "My husband, you know, he had all the testing and stuff, and there was nothing wrong with him," one woman recalls. "It was all me. The problems were all mine. The guilt I felt! Kids love my husband—he just attracts them. I almost left him because I felt so guilty that I was the reason he wouldn't be having kids. And then the miscarriage—that was me, too. He finally convinced me that he was happy with me, and that he wouldn't be happy without me."

For couples who never find out what caused their infertility, facing another unsolved mystery with the miscarriage is just too much: "Is it something hereditary? Should I be angry with my parents?"

LETTING YOURSELF OFF THE HOOK

Most women feel guilty about losing a pregnancy, even if they don't talk about their feelings. Although it's natural to wonder why you had a miscarriage, it's important to realize that it was not your fault. Most miscarriages have no known cause, or they have a genetic component and would have occurred no matter what you did or did not do. It is doubtful that you could have done anything to prevent it. Miscarriages are not caused by working too hard, having sex, carrying heavy packages, being too stressed, not eating properly, sleeping too little, or exercising.

If you're feeling guilty and afraid that you caused your miscarriage, talk to your doctor or midwife about it. Your provider will likely tell you that there was no specific cause, and that the miscarriage was going to happen no matter what you were doing. Another way to deal with feelings of guilt is to educate yourself about miscarriage, including possible contributing factors. The resources listed at the end of the book may be helpful.

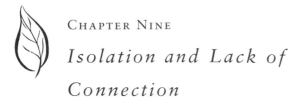

CHAPTER NINE

Isolation and Lack of
Connection

HUMAN BEINGS NATURALLY STRIVE TO FEEL CONNECTED TO
other people and the larger world. Feeling alone is very difficult for most people. Unfortunately, this feeling is all too
familiar to women who miscarry after infertility treatments. The combined effect of miscarriage and infertility
can leave women feeling profoundly isolated, sometimes
even despite the presence of loving family and friends.

Western culture does not have many healthy outlets for
women to express and acknowledge their grief after a miscarriage. Some other cultures do, however. In an article in
the *New York Times Magazine,* American writer Peggy
Orenstein describes her experience of having a miscarriage
while living in Japan. In mourning her loss, she learned of
that culture's special care of women who miscarry. Orenstein was directed to a Buddhist temple in Tokyo, where
she found dozens of small statues of infants. They were
brightly dressed and had colorful pinwheels and vases of
flowers at their sides. Their hands were clasped in prayer,
and their faces were serene. These statues, symbolizing the
short lives of miscarried fetuses, were offerings to Jizo,
an enlightened being who watches over the lost babies.

Women come to the temple to make an offering on behalf of their own lost fetus.

For some women, participating in such a ritual—akin to going to a cemetery to visit a lost relative—can be very soothing. It can make the miscarriage more "real" by commemorating the child who was lost. Not all women find this comforting, but some certainly benefit. In lieu of a cultural ritual such as visiting a Japanese temple, individual rituals such as planting a tree or making a memory book can be healing.

FEELING ISOLATED AND STIGMATIZED

Some women feel isolated and stigmatized because they don't have a child and can't share in other women's stories of pregnancy and childbirth. While their friends are busy talking about their pregnancies, births, and cute kids, these women hesitate to bring up the tough issues they're dealing with—infertility treatments that aren't working or pregnancies that were lost. This makes the feeling of being alone much more pronounced. "It's so disheartening because no one knows how this feels but me," says one woman. "I can't get pregnant again like other people can." Another says, "It makes me feel like because we don't have a baby, we aren't as important as other people."

Women also express dismay at feeling like the bearer of bad news. "I feel like a broken record. I'm always telling bad news. I never have good news to tell." This can exacerbate the feeling of being alone.

FEELING ALONE IN THE HOSPITAL

Women who are admitted to the hospital for a D & C after a miscarriage may be placed on the maternity unit. Hearing babies cry in the nursery or in other women's rooms can be heart-wrenching, which contributes to the feeling of isolation and stigmatization. "I was in the hospital for the D & C, and the nurses didn't come to my room," one woman recalls. "I guess they didn't want anything to do with me because I didn't have a baby." Another woman says, "The nurse would come in and say, 'Did you just have your baby?' and I would just cry and say I lost my baby. That made it so much harder."

"NO ONE HAS HAD THIS EXPERIENCE BUT ME"

Do you know other women who have had a miscarriage after infertility? If so, perhaps you have someone to talk to who can understand your grief and sadness. Most of the women we spoke to did not know anyone else who had had a similar experience. One woman commented, "You feel like you're all alone, and of course where I live, I am all alone because I'm the only one who ever went through this that I know of."

Even women who have supportive friends and family don't necessarily feel connected to them during the first few weeks after the miscarriage. "I'm lucky I have a supportive family that allowed me to cry all the time. I'd be having a fine day, and then suddenly I'd be crying. It went on for weeks. No one could help me," one woman says. Another remembers, "I pretty much shut everybody out of my life because no one could say anything to make me happy or make me feel better, so I just dealt with it by myself. I didn't feel like my husband understood, either. It didn't bother him like it did me, because he wasn't the one who was pregnant. He wasn't the one who lost it. I should give him more credit than that, but that's just how I felt."

CONNECTING AGAIN

It's normal to feel alone in your experience. After all, you're the one going through it. It was your body that had the infertility treatments, became pregnant, and went through the miscarriage. The feeling of being alone in your grief will probably last awhile, and then you'll want to talk to people again, let your loved ones back into your life, and perhaps do something to honor your lost baby. These suggestions may help you move from isolation to connection:

　Tell your family members and friends that you need some time to deal with what has happened. Let them know that you love them but you can't be your old self right now. Remember that it's not up to them to decide how long you should grieve.

🌿 Do something to acknowledge that your pregnancy happened. Many women find it helpful to put together a memory book or journal that includes hospital identity bracelets, ultrasound pictures, appointment cards, and anything else you have from the pregnancy. You might want to write about what happened. Mark down the important dates from the pregnancy, such as the positive pregnancy test, the first prenatal visit, and the date of the miscarriage.

🌿 Some women find it helpful to purchase something that will remind them of the pregnancy they lost. For example, you can buy a birthstone ring or pin to commemorate the month the baby would have been born.

🌿 Plant a tree in the baby's memory, or express your feelings through art. Write a poem or story, keep a journal, or paint a picture. All these things can be helpful, so consider doing one or more of them.

🌿 If you were placed on the maternity unit in the hospital and had a difficult experience, consider writing to the hospital administrator about how uncomfortable this made you feel. Suggest that the hospital's policy be changed so that other women won't have to go through a similar experience. By doing something to help others, you may feel less alone and more connected with other women.

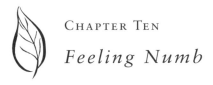

CHAPTER TEN

Feeling Numb

MANY WOMEN REPORT FEELING NUMB FOR A TIME AFTER their miscarriage. This might mean not being able to enjoy much of anything and feeling like you're "sleep-walking" through your life. You take no joy from things you usually love. You don't want to entertain, listen to music, spend time with friends, or even eat your favorite foods. It is similar to the way many people feel during depression. The feeling may last for a few days or weeks, then gradually lift.

Some women find the sense of numbness comforting, because feeling nothing at all is easier than feeling the pain. If you "shut down," however, it can be frightening for your partner, who may find it hard to help you or feel close to you.

CRYING AND SLEEPING

Immediately after a miscarriage, many women just go through the motions of life. They cry and sleep. They don't want to talk to anyone or even leave the house: "In the beginning I cried all the time. I couldn't go down the baby aisle at the supermarket. My soul was empty. My body was empty." "I sat in the house for two weeks. I wanted to be alone, I didn't want to talk to anyone. It was even hard for me to go to church." "I was just numb and I don't know that I had any real feelings at first. It took me an hour or so after the doctor told me before I started crying. I was in disbelief that it was happening. Once I started crying, I couldn't stop. Then I relived it each day. I felt exhausted and low and sad." "It was like a funeral, that miscarriage. I felt really bad for a few months, then I saw a counselor who helped me." "I guess I was in a major depression. I couldn't leave the house. It was just really, really hard. The breakthrough for me was finding out the reason for the miscarriage. That God wasn't trying to punish me. Then all I could think about was trying again."

GRIEVING IN YOUR OWN WAY
IN YOUR OWN TIME

Feeling numb is a normal reaction to the overwhelming sadness of a miscarriage after infertility. You shouldn't worry that it's wrong to feel so bad. It's important to allow yourself to feel the grief in your own way, to express it when you are able to do so, and then to move on.

Most women who felt numb after their miscarriage say that the only thing that helps is time. You may feel numb for a few days or a few weeks. If you're able to openly

YOUR LOSS IS REAL

Some people may tell you that you should be happy and grateful that at least you became pregnant. While it might be true that your pregnancy was a good sign that you're capable of becoming pregnant, it is also true that you have suffered a loss, and you deserve as much time as you need to grieve that loss.

express your grief and sadness, it should gradually start to lessen. Don't be afraid to cry, be angry, punch a pillow, scream, and yell. Do whatever you need to do to start feeling better.

If you're still feeling numb after a month and you're not able to function in your day-to-day activities, seek counseling from a therapist or consider joining a bereavement support group. Talking to other people who have experienced loss can help you resolve your own grief.

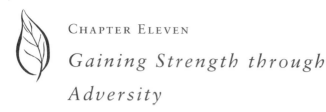

CHAPTER ELEVEN

Gaining Strength through Adversity

WHILE MANY OF THE EMOTIONS CONNECTED TO MISCAR-
riage after infertility are painful and negative, the experience can lead to some positive outcomes. Women who have
been through this experience describe closer personal rela-
tionships, deepened spiritual feelings, and increased
personal strength.

STRONGER RELATIONSHIP WITH A SPOUSE
OR PARTNER

Your relationship with your spouse or significant
other may become stronger as you go through this difficult experience together. For some couples, a very strong
bond develops because they see themselves as the only two
people who really know what the loss of their potential son
or daughter means. Others become closer through the
sense of working together to overcome a crisis.

"I said to my husband, 'We can't let this ruin our marriage,' and we didn't," one woman notes. Another says,
"In a funny way it made my marriage stronger. We got
through it. We got through it together."

For some women, the bonding with their spouse was the only positive outcome from the miscarriage, but it was essential to their grief resolution.

STRONGER RELATIONSHIP WITH GOD

Although many women express anger with God about having to experience infertility and miscarriage, some say their relationship with God is stronger because of the miscarriage: "I pray over this, and I'm closer to God now. I have to put myself in God's hands."

Miscarriage can put you in touch with your spirituality as you try to understand the role of adversity in your life and the lessons you may learn because of it. One woman reflects, "When I look back on it, I think the whole experience has taken me to a new level in my relationship with God. It has strengthened me and has somehow made me a better person, a humbler person."

BECOMING STRONGER

The experience of miscarriage makes some women feel stronger as individuals. Before a miscarriage, many women are timid around doctors, following doctors' orders without questioning them. But this often changes after a miscarriage. Many women begin taking charge of their own lives and healthcare. One woman says, "I used to hold doctors up on a pedestal, and I was afraid to ask them anything or question anything they said. But going through all of this, I found out that they are human, too. Now I feel like I know my body better than they do, so I can question them and say, 'No, that's not what's going on,' or 'No, that's not what I want.'"

For other women, miscarriage teaches them that they'll never have complete control over their lives, and that they need to be more adaptable. "I'm not as depressed as I used to be," one woman says. "I look at the other things in my life. The good things. I know that I need to be upbeat. I push the sadness away. It made me a stronger person." Another woman notes, "Going through this miscarriage has helped me to better understand how precious life is." One woman joined a support group and learned about the trials other people were going through. "Worse things have happened to people, much worse things," she says. "I try to stay positive."

FINDING PEACE

Most experiences do have some positive aspects, but you might not be able to focus on those until your active grieving is over. If a positive thought pops into your mind about your miscarriage, don't worry that you are betraying your lost child. Every bad experience can have a positive side, and thinking about this can help you resolve your grief.

Most people who have lived through difficult and traumatic experiences travel the same road of grief, sadness, anger, acceptance, and, finally, hope for the future. While you may not believe it just yet, you will find peace again in your life. It helps if you can allow yourself to feel all your emotions. Grief has no time limit, and everyone experiences it in her own way, but eventually you will feel better. You will enjoy life again, and you will come to terms with the miscarriage you experienced after infertility treatments.

Resources

The following Web sites provide information about infertility, pregnancy, miscarriage, and grieving. Although these addresses were accurate at the time of publication, please note that Web sites change frequently.

www.americaninfertility.org

The American Infertility Association has information from reproductive professionals as well as a message board for patients' questions.

www.babycenter.com

BabyCenter provides information and advertisements about pregnancy and infancy. It also has some useful information about miscarriage.

www.chem-tox.com/infertility

Two researchers from University of South Florida have developed this site about environmental causes of infertility.

www.compassionatefriends.org

The Compassionate Friends is a support group for

people who have had miscarriages or stillbirths or experienced the death of a child.

www.earlypath.com

A medical doctor who is a pathologist provides information on early pregnancy loss.

www.fertilityplus.org

Written "by patients for patients," this site contains information about all aspects of infertility, including miscarriage.

www.inciid.org

The InterNational Council on Infertility Information Dissemination provides information and support for people dealing with infertility and pregnancy loss.

www.ivf.com/misc.html

The story of a woman who suffered a miscarriage after having in vitro fertilization is included on this site, which is the homepage for a group of infertility specialists in Georgia.

www.nationalshareoffice.com

SHARE Pregnancy and Infant Loss Support is a not-for-profit organization for families who have lost a pregnancy or an infant.

www.parents.com/articles/pregnancy/1225.jsp?page=3

This article discusses possible causes of miscarriage.

www.resolve.org

RESOLVE: The National Infertility Association offers educational materials and support to families with infertility.

www.womens-health.co.uk/miscarr.htm

This British Web site contains an article about miscarriage written by a doctor.

Bibliography

Brier, Norman. "Understanding and Managing the Emotional Reactions to a Miscarriage." *Obstetrics and Gynecology* 93 (1): 151-55 (1999).

Cote-Arsenault, Denise, and Dianne Morrison-Beedy. "Women's Voices Reflecting Changed Expectations for Pregnancy after Perinatal Loss." *Journal of Nursing Scholarship* 3 (3): 239-44 (2001).

Cramer, Daniel W., and Lauren A. Wise. "The Epidemiology of Recurrent Pregnancy Loss." *Seminars in Reproductive Medicine* 18 (4): 331-39 (2000).

Cuisinier, Marianne, Herman Janssen, Chris deGraauw, Siem Bakker, and Cal Hoogduin. "Pregnancy Following Miscarriage: Course of Grief and Some Determining Factors." *Journal of Psychosomatic Obstetrics and Gynecology* 17 (3): 168-74 (1996).

Englehard, Iris M., Marcel A. van den Hout, and Arnoud Arntz. "Posttraumatic Stress Disorder after Pregnancy Loss." *General Hospital Psychiatry* 23 (2): 62-66 (2001).

Freda, Margaret Comerford, Kit Devine, and Carrie F. Semelsberger. "The Lived Experience of Miscarriage after Infertility." *MCN, The American Journal of Maternal Child Nursing* 28 (1): 16-23 (2003).

Lee, Christina, and Pauline Slade. "Miscarriage as a Traumatic Event: A Review of the Literature and New Implications for Intervention." *Journal of Psychosomatic Research* 40 (3): 235-44 (1996).

Lukse, Michelle P., and Nicholas A. Vacc. "Grief, Depression, and Coping in Women Undergoing Infertility Treatment." *Obstetrics and Gynecology* 93 (2): 245-51 (1999).

Mori, Emi, Toshihide Nadaoka, Yukiko Morioka, and Hidekazu Saito. "Anxiety of Infertile Women undergoing IVF-ET: Relation to the Grief Process." *Gynecologic Obstetric Investigation* 44 (3): 157-62 (1997).

Orenstein, Peggy. "Mourning My Miscarriage." *New York Times Magazine*, 21 April 2002, 38.

Pezeshki, Kevin, Joseph Feldman, Daniel E. Stein, Susan M. Lobel, and Richard V. Grazi. "Bleeding and Spontaneous Abortion after Therapy for Infertility." *Fertility and Sterility* 74 (3): 504-48 (2000).

Prettyman, R. J., C. J. Cordle, and G. D. Cook. "A Three-Month Follow-Up of Psychological Morbidity after Early Miscarriage." *British Journal of Medical Psychology* 66: 363-72 (1993).

Schoener, Claudia J., and Lois W. Krysa. "The Comfort and Discomfort of Infertility." *Journal of Obstetric Gynecologic and Neonatal Nursing* 25 (2): 167-72 (1996).

Slade, Pauline. "Predicting the Psychological Impact of Miscarriage." *Journal of Reproductive and Infant Psychology* 12: 5-16 (1994).

Speroff, Leon, Robert H. Glass, and Nathan G. Kase. "Recurrent Pregnancy Loss." In *Clinical Gynecologic Endocrinology and Infertility,* 6th edition. Edited by Leon Speroff, Robert H. Glass, and Nathan G. Kase. Philadelphia: Lippincott, Williams and Wilkins, 1999.

Swanson, Kristin M. "Predicting Depressive Symptoms after Miscarriage: A Path Analysis Based on the Lazarus Paradigm." *Journal of Women's Health and Gender-Based Medicine* 9 (2):191-206 (2000).

Syme, G. B. "Facing the Unacceptable: The Emotional Response to Infertility." *Human Reproduction* 12 (11): 183-87 (1997).

Turner, J. J., G. M. Flannelly, M. Wingfield, J. J. Rasmussen, R. Ryan, S. Cullen, R. Maguire, and M. Stronge. "Miscarriage Clinic: An Audit of the First Year." *British Journal of Obstetrics and Gynecology* 98: 306-08 (1998).

About the Authors

DR. MARGARET COMERFORD FREDA is a professor in the Department of Obstetrics & Gynecology and Women's Health, Albert Einstein College of Medicine, Montefiore Medical Center, Bronx, New York. She also serves as director of patient education programs for the department. Dr. Freda is a consultant for nursing at the National March of Dimes Birth Defects Foundation and the chair of the National March of Dimes Nurse Advisory Council. In addition, Dr. Freda is the editor of *MCN, The American Journal of Maternal Child Nursing.*

Dr. Freda received her diploma in nursing from Misericordia Hospital School of Nursing, her BSN from Stony Brook University, her master's degree in nursing from New York University, and her doctorate in health education from Columbia University. She has spent her entire professional career working in women's health. Her research has focused on preterm birth prevention and on women's health education needs.

Dr. Freda has published more than fifty articles in professional journals, and she is frequently invited to speak at nursing and medical conferences. She has received several noteworthy awards, including the Distinguished

Professional Service Award from the Association of Women's Health, Obstetric and Neonatal Nurses (AWHONN), the Woman of Distinction Award from the March of Dimes, the First National Award for Excellence in Nursing Research from AWHONN, the Patient Care Award for Excellence in Patient Education from the American Academy of Family Physicians, the Maternal Child Nurse of the Year Award from the Greater New York Chapter March of Dimes, and the Nursing Research Recognition Award from Molloy College.

Dr. Freda has developed patient education booklets and videotapes that are distributed nationally. Her book for nurses, *Perinatal Patient Education: A Practical Guide with Education Handouts for Patients*, was published in 2002 by Lippincott and received the American Journal of Nursing Book of the Year Award. Dr. Freda responds online to the public's questions on pregnancy at www. pampers.com, the Web site for the Proctor and Gamble Pampers Parenting Institute, of which she is a board member.

CARRIE F. SEMELSBERGER graduated from the School of Nursing at Stony Brook University in 2003. She is currently a neonatal intensive care nurse. She was formerly an elementary school teacher, having received a baccalaureate degree from Towson University in Maryland. Ms. Semelsberger was treated for infertility and subsequently suffered a miscarriage. Her experiences and inability to find appropriate reading material were the impetus for this book.

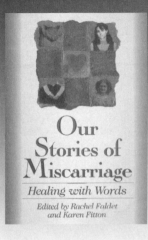

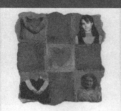

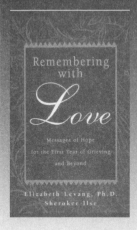

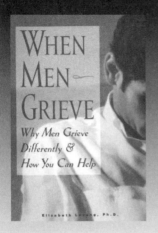